Surviving

Dengue

Fever

A Personal Day-by-Day Account
of the Symptoms, Treatment and
Long-term Aftereffects

G. Roebuck

ISBN-13: 978-1475240214

ISBN-10: 147524021X

Dedicated to the scientists and
researchers striving to find a vaccine for
Dengue Fever, Zika and other tropical
diseases

CONTENTS

v

Preface

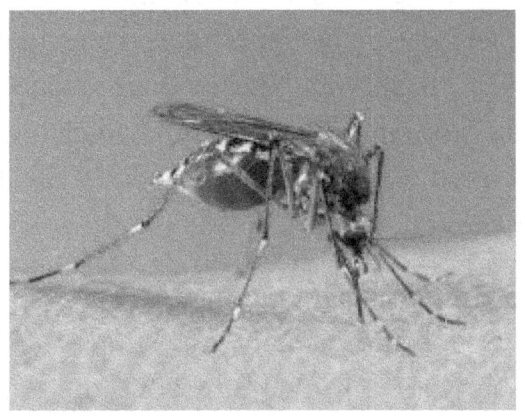

As a fit and healthy world traveler, I was used to taking sensible precautions against malaria, mosquito bites and other diseases. I certainly never expected to contract Dengue (pronounced DENgee) fever, especially on the very civilized island of Tahiti, but unfortunately I did.

This book is my day-by-day account of the symptoms and treatment I experienced, along with simple information about the disease in layman's terms. It was carefully written to help anyone diagnosed with Dengue Fever, or their carer, to know what to expect, how to alleviate the symptoms, and how long the effects of Dengue Fever were likely to last. It also includes some facts about the similar Zika virus, which was declared a "global public health emergency" by the WHO.

Once I had been diagnosed with Dengue Fever, I had many questions, so I researched information about the virus on the internet. The information I found was either in highly technical medical language or blasé generalized information suggesting that Dengue Fever was no more serious than flu and would be over in a matter of days. There was frustrating little useful information available to answer my many questions such as:

How did I catch Dengue Fever?

Is it Dengue, Chikungunya or Zika?

How long would the fever last?

Why did painkillers not alleviate the headache?

Why was taking aspirin and ibuprofen dangerous for Dengue patients?

How long would the rash last?

Why were my hands and feet red and swollen?

Why did my fingers and feet suddenly shed their skin two months after contracting Dengue Fever?

Was the crippling pain and stiffness in my knees and ankles related to Dengue Fever?

Although I received excellent medical care in hospital in Sydney, Australia, whenever I asked specific questions about my symptoms the reply generally was, "We don't really know. We haven't nursed anyone with Dengue Fever before". Even specialists from the Sydney Centre for Tropical Diseases led me to believe that the rash would only last for 24 hours and then the worst of the infection would be over. In reality that was far from the truth. I was certainly not prepared for the lengthy recovery time needed. Three months after being diagnosed I was still suffering from peeling skin and stiff, painful joints.

Despite there being an estimated 100 million cases of Dengue Fever worldwide every year, there is no true step-by-step account of what to expect as a sufferer, or any information available to prepare me for the fact that it would take months before I was free from the painful side effects.

Many websites gave a list of symptoms of Dengue Fever that a patient may or may not suffer, with the reassurance that they would only last up to 10 days. Symptoms were vague, partly due to the fact that there are five different strains of Dengue Fever. I discovered that Dengue

Fever affected different people in different ways and to different degrees.

As a previously health and active adult, the only way I knew whether a symptom was Dengue related or not was by comparing my symptoms with my husband, who had also earlier contracted Dengue Fever.

The combination of lack of expertise from medical practitioners outside the tropics and vague general information about Dengue on the internet inspired me to write this personal account of what Dengue Fever was really like. By listing it as a day-by-day and week-by week account, I hope it will offer relevant information to reassure those suffering from Dengue, or nursing someone with the disease, that the strange things going on in their body were probably still the results of the fever, even months after the fever itself was over.

To further reinforce the information, I have included comparable information from my husband's experience of Dengue Fever as a second case study. He contracted Dengue Fever earlier than I did and his symptoms were quite different in some ways to my own. His experience helps to offer a broader experience of what Dengue Fever sufferers are likely to go through, especially during the long and painful recovery process.

By knowing what to expect, Dengue Fever sufferers can plan their life accordingly, taking into account the tiredness, lethargy, painful joints and lack of mobility that persists for months while you recover.

This book also touches on the difference between Zika, Chikungunya and Dengue fever which are all spread by the Aedes Aegypti mosquito and have similar initial symptoms.

Background Information

Readers should note that I am a fit and healthy woman in my mid-50s with no serious health issues. My husband is of similar age, again with no major health issues apart from slightly raised blood pressure which he takes medication for.

We had vacationed in Tahiti where my husband was diagnosed with Dengue Fever. I did not get any symptoms until we reached Australia and was touring New South Wales, about 7 days later.

Surviving Dengue Fever

**A Personal Day-by-Day Account
of the Symptoms, Treatment and
Long-term Aftereffects**

FACT: Dengue Fever can kill you

FICTION: Dengue Fever only lasts 2 weeks

Day 1

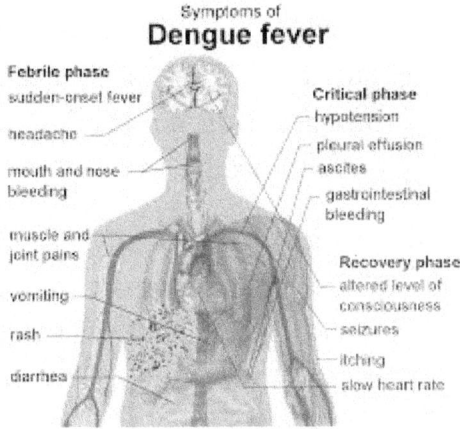

The first symptom of Dengue Fever for me was a terrible headache. I suffer from occasional migraines and this headache took the form of the usual pain over my right eye and a feeling of nausea. However, it was accompanied by an unusual stabbing headache up the back of my head and in the bone behind my left ear.

I took my usual prescription migraine medication which was a sachet of Migramax (900mg aspirin and 10mg metoclopramide (INN) hydrochloride EP in a water solution) plus one Naramig tablet (naratriptan). This stopped the migraine pain at the front of my head but had no effect at all on the stabbing pain at the back of my head.

The pain came intermittently, from 30 seconds to five minutes apart. It would hit in a series of jabs that struck up the back of my head with such force that I literally jumped each time.

During the day, the nausea came and went but I managed to eat something and was not physically sick. We were driving all day but when we reached our hotel for the evening I felt tired, weak and sick and headed straight for bed.

During the night I woke up shivering with cold. I piled a thick feather duvet on top of the bed which made no difference, so eventually I got up and put on several layers of clothing. Still my teeth chattered with cold. I slept fitfully, mainly due to the stabbing headache, nausea and cold chills.

Case Study 2

In contrast, my husband's first symptoms of Dengue Fever were totally different to mine. As he contracted Dengue Fever first, we had no way of knowing what to expect.

He awoke with a slight headache and took a painkiller (paracetamol) which seemed to treat it. Later in the morning he was on the telephone and at the end of the phone call, almost without warning, he was suddenly and violently sick. Thinking he had a stomach bug, he lay down on the bed and slept for most of the day. When he awoke he had a high temperature and felt nauseous and generally unwell.

That night he tossed and turned with a temperature of 104°F (40°C) and possibly higher, which I knew was dangerous. I sponged him down with a cool flannel from time to time and eventually gave him a tepid shower during the night to try to lower his temperature. Every time he sipped water he was sick again, which made it difficult to hold down fluids or painkillers to control the fever.

Day 2

In my case, finding myself in a strange country with no doctor, I decided to go to the local A&E department of the hospital to see if they could give me stronger painkillers for the headache, which I thought was probably just an ear infection requiring antibiotics.

After checking in, the nurse took my details and I informed them that I had just arrived from Tahiti. She gave me ibuprofen to help ease the head and ear pain while I waited for the doctor. Within 30 minutes the stabbing pain at the back of my ear had finally eased.

The doctor thoroughly examined me and suspected encephalitis. He advised that I should continue taking my medication for migraine, but if I got any stiffness in the neck or if the symptoms worsened I should seek medical attention again.

With the headache and ear pain now gone, I managed to eat breakfast and continued on our long car journey to Sydney. Unfortunately, by lunchtime the stabbing pain was back worse than ever, so I took more ibuprofen which seemed to be the only thing that eased the pain. What I did not know until later, when Dengue Fever was diagnosed, was that **taking ibuprofen is extremely dangerous for Dengue sufferers and could even be fatal.**

I slept fitfully again that night but the next morning felt weak, nauseous and ill. I was able to walk but had little appetite and all I wanted to do was lie down.

Case Study 2

Unlike me, my husband's early symptoms of Dengue Fever were a high temperature, fever and sickness. We visited the local doctor and after a thorough examination, he pronounced that he suspected that my husband had

Dengue Fever. It was hard to determine this, as the symptoms are similar to the less serious Zika virus which is also rife in Tahiti and causes general malaise, skin rash, fever and muscle pain. Next step was to visit a clinic where a nurse took a blood test. That same afternoon we had a phone call saying that the blood test confirmed that the symptoms were due to Dengue Fever.

In my husband's case, the main problem was a very high fever, although he did not sweat. The recommended treatment was 1g (1000mg) paracetamol every four hours and drinking plenty of fluids. This proved a problem as he continued to be sick every time any food or water was consumed. By evening he did manage to keep down a thin piece of dry bread and some paracetamol.

His temperature continued to register 104°F (40°C) and to try to control it in the tropical heat, he sat in the unheated pool beneath a shady umbrella. The other aid which I would highly recommend was a Frogg Toggs Chilly Pad Cooling Towel. These hyper-evaporative synthetic cloths hold an enormous amount of water and remain cool to the touch for hours. It was ideal for my husband to use during the nighttime as he could sleep with it draped across his forehead to help keep him cool.

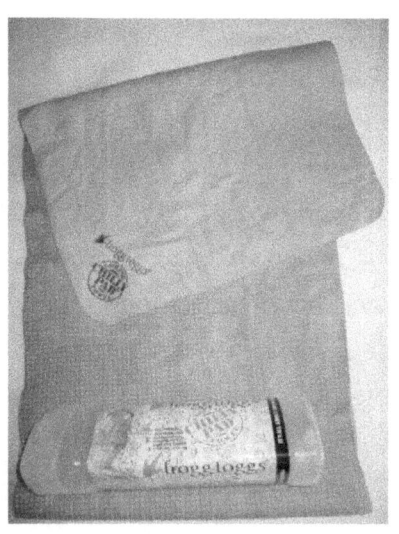

Day 3

I spent the third day resting, eating a little, and trying to control the stabbing headache and ear pain. I felt generally tired, weak and nauseous although the fever appeared to have passed.

Case Study 2

In my husband's case he still had an exceptionally high temperature which he tried to reduce with paracetamol and the use of the Frogg Toggs Chilly Pad on his upper chest and forehead. He mostly slept, and ate nothing as he felt nauseous. He continued to be sick when he drank water, making dehydration a problem.

Day 4

With no sign of improvement after four days of pain and weakness, I decided to go to the A&E department at the local hospital to see if they could relieve my symptoms. By now I was feeling decidedly weak, could hardly walk, and felt increasingly dizzy and nauseous while still being plagued by the stabbing head and ear pain. I had also had slight bleeding from the gums which was very unusual for me.

During the initial examination by a nurse, I apparently had a "funny turn" and passed out for a short time. When I came to I was on a trolley heading for a CT brain scan. This did not show any edema, hemorrhage or abnormalities. Next, the doctor examined and questioned me and I again reiterated that I had been staying in Tahiti, just in case that had any bearing on my sickness.

The blood test results showed that I had an alarmingly low blood count of platelets (thrombocytopenia) with a count of 75 instead of the normal 250; low white blood cell count (leukopenia/neutropenia) with a WCC of 2.0, and there was concern about my liver function. The doctor decided to admit me to the ward for observation while they took further blood tests and sent them away for culture to diagnose exactly what the underlying disease was. At this stage they were considering several tropical diseases including malaria, dengue and Zika.

I was put on a fluid drip containing electrolytes as I was very dehydrated. I was also given an anti-emetic drip to control the nausea, and painkillers for the headache. However, ibuprofen was forbidden as I then learnt that it could worsen internal bleeding and leakage from the veins.

Case Study 2

In my husband's case, sleeping and drinking plenty of fluids along with paracetamol were the only treatments available to counter the nausea and fever that he experienced. He felt extremely tired, generally ill all over his body and was unable to stand or walk more than a few steps.

He developed a fine red rash around his upper chest and on his lower legs which he kept cool using the Froggy Togg towel.

Day 5

I slept for much of the day in hospital and felt listless and ill. I managed to eat small amounts of light food at each meal and was encouraged to drink plenty of water. Blood tests were taken each morning to monitor platelets, which kept going down. Body temperature showed a continuing mild fever.

I remained on a drip of fluids and was given an anti-emetic to control nausea. I also took painkillers, although the striking headache was now much less painful.

I developed an extreme tenderness on my skin, fingertips and feet. My fingers became so sensitive that I could only loosely hold a fork or spoon and certainly could not take the screw cap off my water bottle. I also noticed I had a tender scalp when washing my hair.

The soles of my feet were so tender that I could only wear the softest slippers to walk to the bathroom or when I took a short stroll in the hospital grounds. The pain was so extreme that when I stepped out of the shower onto the edge of the floor mat I was in agony.

Case Study 2

By day 5, nausea and sickness were still a problem for my husband and he spent much of the day asleep or just lying on the bed. He was still unable to eat anything. When he stood up he swayed and was unable to walk to the bathroom in a straight line. His general discomfort and fever made it difficult for him to sleep at night so he took Melatonin which helped. The fever and high temperature seemed to be receding but he still felt weak and unwell.

The fine measles-like red rash he developed the day before appeared to spread further on his body and legs.

Day 6

The results of my blood tests came back negative for malaria, according to the doctor, who always wore a mask when visiting and examining me. He still suspected Dengue Fever, but wanted to have it confirmed just to be sure. Another morning blood test was taken and the results showed a further drop in platelets to 37 and a decrease in neutrophils to 0.8. There was a continued worsening of my liver function throughout my stay.

A urine sample showed the presence of an E.coli infection, so I was put on a drip of antibiotics (tazocin). This was apparently due to a concern about the risk of neutropaenic sepsis which can become life-threatening. With such a low blood count, obviously my immune system was weakened as it fought the Dengue Fever infection. The doctors emphasized the importance of preventing any further infection in my vulnerable state. A blood transfusion was considered but held off in the hope of the blood cell count improving naturally.

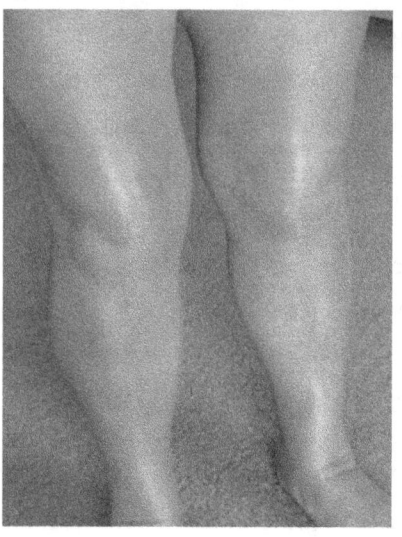

Later in the day I developed a dark red rash on my legs and feet. It was very fine and bumpy, a little like a measles rash or an allergic drug reaction. It became itchy when hot. The best relief was a bag of ice wrapped in a towel which I used night and day to keep my legs cool and comfortable. My arms also developed a purple blotchy pattern under the skin due to vein seepage.

Case Study 2

In my husband's case, the fever finally receded and he ate his first mouthful of food in almost a week – scrambled egg! He was still very weak on his legs and could not stand or walk very far. He was also still suffering from slight dizziness and wanted to sleep in the day as well as all night long. He had no interest in reading or watching TV, but seemed to be slowly improving as the fever had finally abated.

This for him was the sixth day of sickness. The palms of his hands had suddenly turned bright red and were very sensitive to the touch. The rash continued to cover his lower legs. The soles of his feet were also ultra-sensitive.

Day 7

Finally, a week after the first symptoms appeared, the blood tests taken on Day 4 confirmed I had Dengue Fever. As there is currently no cure, just treatment for the symptoms, there was nothing more to be done. Morning blood tests showed a continued decline in cell count and liver function.

The antibiotics were stopped as there was a possibility that they were aggravating the fiery red rash on my legs, which now looked like a bad case of sunburn.

The nausea had passed and I was back to eating normally and still drinking lots of water. I slept part of the day but generally felt brighter and was able to concentrate and read for a while.

I was visited by a consultant specialist from the Sydney Centre for Tropical Diseases who was very informative and helpful. He warned me that **it was unwise for me to ever visit an area where Dengue Fever was prevalent as a second attack of Dengue would be far more serious.** This unfortunately ruled out travelling to much of Asia, Central and South America. He explained that there is a much greater risk of developing the more serious Dengue Hemorrhagic Fever for anyone who had antibodies from a previous Dengue virus. The risk of Hemorrhagic Fever is also higher if you are female, Caucasian or under the age of 12.

This is one way in which Dengue Fever differs from Zika. Once a person has been infected with the Zika virus, they are immunized from future infection. In the case of Dengue Fever, however, the antibody dependent enhancement means that contracting a second type of Dengue actually raises the risk of triggering life-threatening hemorrhagic fever.

Case Study 2

After a week, my husband continued to feel drowsy and weak and spent most of the day asleep in a soft, comfortable chair with his feet supported on a soft cushion. His hands were red and supersensitive and he had trouble holding a fork or spoon to eat anything. He had no appetite and the soles of his feet were too sensitive to rest on the floor. His body was also sensitive to touch.

Day 8

Blood tests continued to show decreasing levels of platelets and white blood cells. However, my temperature and blood pressure were normal. I felt generally weak and still had extremely tender feet, so it was very difficult to walk. The rash on my legs was gradually reducing from the top of my leg towards the knee and resembled red knee-high socks.

Case Study 2

In my husband's case, his appetite and strength were slowly returning. He was able to walk a short distance but still had the eggplant-colored rash on his lower legs. He felt weak and disorientated and could not concentrate on anything for very long. Everything seemed to taste peculiar, even coffee, and his saliva seemed to be thick and nasty. Sucking mints was a help. So far he had lost 11 pounds in weight.

Day 9

Finally there was a slight improvement in the morning blood tests which showed slightly higher platelets and improved white blood cell count. However there was still concern about my liver function and I was advised to avoid alcohol until more normal levels had been reached.

After a final warning about avoiding any area in future where Dengue Fever was likely, I was released from hospital. I was generally weak, tired and still had a nasty rash from the knee to the foot which looked like dark red knee socks.

Case Study 2

In my husband's case, after nine days he was slowly getting back to normal but was very tired and lethargic. The rash was receding, leaving just a dark shadow on the lower leg. However the soles of his feet, like mine, were extremely sensitive, making it difficult to wear shoes or walk far.

Days 10-13

Once home from hospital, I continued to improve slowly day by day. I had lost about five pounds in weight. The main problems were my tender fingers and inflamed soles of my feet. This meant that I could not walk far. I still wore soft slippers rather than wearing shoes or walking barefoot on the hard floor tiles.

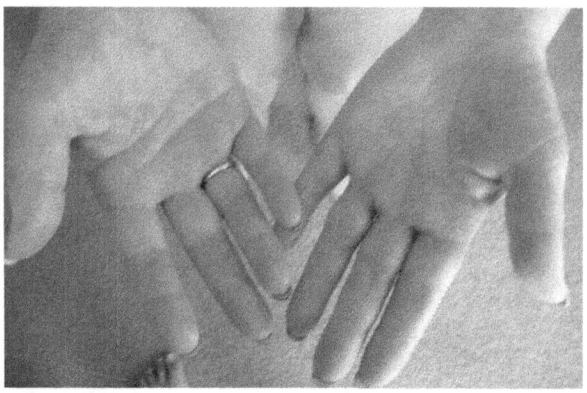

I tired very easily and was generally lethargic but my appetite was good and there no specific pain.

Case Study 2

Although physically improving, my husband suffered periods of irrational anxiety and worry that was total unlike him. Clearly it was a side effect of Dengue Fever as I also experienced it a week later in my recovery.

Week 3

Even three weeks after the first symptoms of Dengue Fever I was still easily tired physically. Walking remained slow and painful although I had progressed to wearing sandals. A ten minute walk to the shops, which pre-Dengue was no problem, was still very tiring and I walked very slowly on the return trip.

The effort of stepping up a curb after crossing the road, or even walking up a disabled ramp from the road to the footpath made my thighs ache painfully. Joints become very painful and even slight inclines were physically taxing for my hips and thigh muscles to cope with.

I generally felt very fragile both physically and emotionally when faced with a problem or task. At times I felt worried about the future, which was totally out of character, and on several occasions I lay awake worrying about minor problems that I would normally take in my stride.

Case Study 2

Like me, my husband continued to function with daily tasks but felt extremely fragile. He tired easily and could not walk far before finding his muscles and joints ached.

One day, in the third week of Dengue, he awoke and felt extremely dizzy and could not stand or sit without the world spinning and making him feel disoriented. He found that taking chewable Kwells (hyoscine hydrobromide), an over-the-counter medication normally used for travel sickness, helped alleviate the symptoms and he spent the days sitting reading quietly. Anything further was still out of the question.

Week 4

My feet still had tender spots on the ends of my toes and under the heel. I lacked my normal energy. Walking was still a challenge and even after just a short walk my muscles and joints hurt painfully. I can understand why this disease is known as "Breakbone fever"!

Any gentle physical exercise made my joints begin to hurt, followed by my thighs and hip joints. Even slight inclines or climbing a few steps left my legs aching and my body generally felt tired and weary. When I got up each morning, my ankles and knees were extremely stiff and reluctant to walk. It felt like a sudden onset of arthritis, although I had never suffered from any type of stiffness or pain in the joints before having Dengue Fever. Having researched the topic, I eventually found reference to this being quite normal following Dengue Fever, which was reassuring to know.

Another shock I had this week was that skin from my toes, heels and soles of my feet began to peel. Thick layers came off like old wallpaper, leaving pink, tender skin underneath. Unfortunately, the "frayed edges" of the old skin became dry and hard, catching on socks or bed sheets which was very uncomfortable.

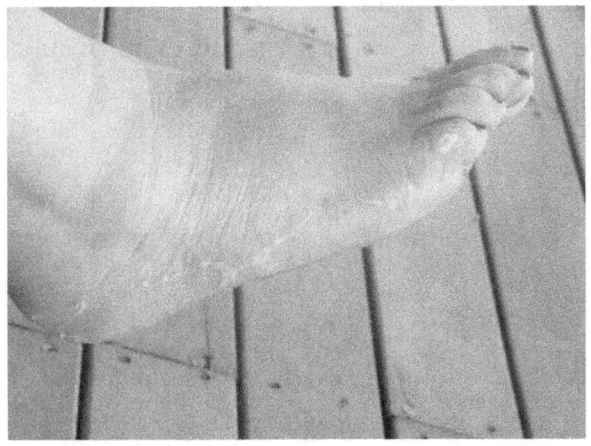

My hands had a similar problem with skin peeling, particularly on the fingertips. They remained tender when I tried to undo bottle tops etc. and looked awful with blotches of frayed skin.

One further strange episode that week was that I became extremely dizzy one day and could not balance or walk. It was like extreme vertigo and I had to catch onto someone's arm or a rail for support. I also felt as if I might faint at times. I took seasickness tablets to ease the symptoms of vertigo, which seemed to help. This lasted for one full day and recurred in a mild form a couple of days later.

Case Study 2

My husband also had a minor recurrence of the dizziness he had had the previous week. It affected his balance and he was unsteady and felt that he would fall over if he was not sat down. Obviously he avoided driving.

The skin on his feet also began to peel off and he experienced the same peeling skin problem on his hands.

Week 5

My feet continued to be tender on the sole, particularly under the heel and around the back of the heel, similar to having pulled a tendon. I learnt to stretch and hold my feet towards my body for a count of 10 before getting up from sleeping or sitting. This helped to lessen the pain when I stood and walk after a period of inactivity.

Slow walking for short distances was OK, but I still needed to hang on to the shopping trolley in supermarkets for support. My legs tire and ached easily and even my shin bones ached after walking. I felt that I had aged about 20 years since catching Dengue Fever.

My knees developed tenderness and pain, particularly when I knelt, even on the bed. They would not support my weight due to the extreme pain.

The skin on my feet continued to peel off in strips.

Case Study 2

My husband was also still suffering with pain in his joints, particularly in his left hip, with sciatica-like pain after sitting. He was still wobbly with vertigo from time to time, especially when bending forward or looking down.

Weeks 6-11

The peeling skin on my hands was finally finished and just small areas remain "frayed" on my feet. My heels still felt tender and inflamed underneath and this was worse after I had walked. My joints were still very stiff and painful in the morning and took a few minutes to loosen up and stop hurting.

At this stage I started taking ibuprofen every day which seems to lessen the inflammation and stiffness compared to when I stopped taking it. The thigh and hip pain were now almost gone and I was able to enjoy longer walks and exercise.

Case Study 2

My husband gradually became more active as his joint pain receded. The vertigo disappeared and he generally felt stronger and recovered his natural energy and joie de vivre. During this finally recovery phase, on a couple of occasions he noticed a sudden shedding of the hair on his head. This was not the usual amount of hair loss after a shower; rather the whole shower stall and every tile in the bathroom were covered in hairs. However, the hair loss stopped as suddenly as it started.

Week 12

I finally felt 99% over Dengue Fever, at last. It took almost three months to recover from when the first symptoms began to show.

I still had tender spots under my heels when I walked, but my thighs, hips and knee joints caused me less pain. I still did not walk as far as I used to as my legs would tire and my joints became achy and stiff the following day, but a 30-45 minute walk for exercise was now possible.

Case Study 2

My husband finally announced that he felt back to normal at last after his bout with Dengue Fever. It took nearly three months for him to recover his energy, strength and ability to concentrate again.

What is Dengue Fever?

Dengue Fever is a mosquito-borne disease which causes a high fever and severe pain in the joints. It is commonly known as "Breakbone fever" due to the pain it causes. An accompanying rash occurs in 50-80% of cases.

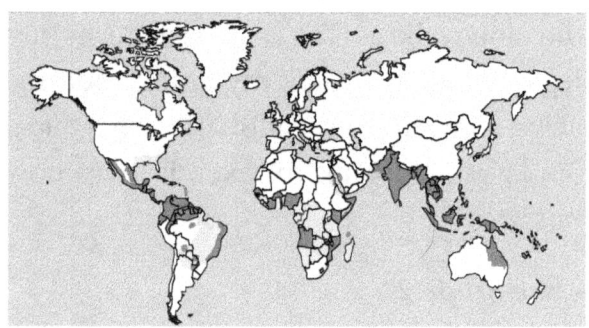

There are currently five strains of Dengue Fever affecting an estimated 50-100 million people every year, according to the World Health Organization (WHO). Other sources calculate that it affects closer to 400 million people every year. Dengue is now endemic in more than 125 countries which lie between latitudes 35°North and 35°South. It is described by WHO as **"the fastest spreading vector-borne viral disease"** with **"epidemic potential"** and **"staggering"** consequences" as it continues to increase.

Dengue Fever is not infectious i.e. it cannot be caught directly from another person. The disease is most commonly transmitted by the female Aedes mosquito, mainly the Aedes Aegypti species which is found most frequently in the tropics and subtropics. The mosquito becomes infected when it bites a person already suffering from Dengue Fever. Once the virus has developed in the mosquito's gut (around 8-10 days) it becomes infected. Although the mosquito suffers no ill effects from the virus, when it bites another human it passes the virus in its saliva to the unsuspecting recipient. Around 4-6 days after infection, the sufferer is likely to show symptoms of the disease.

The virus is carried around the body in white blood cells which respond by producing interferons and cytokines which cause the flu-like symptoms and severe pain in the joints and muscles.

What is Zika?

Zika is similar to Dengue Fever and Chikungunya and all three viruses are carried by the same species of mosquito. Symptoms are similar, with Zika sufferers having a fever, fine red skin rash, joint pain and conjunctivitis or red eyes. They fell generally tired and unwell.

In some people, the symptoms are so mild that they barely know they have the Zika virus while others have headaches and painful muscles along with the other symptoms.

Incubation from the bite form an infected mosquito to developing symptoms is anything from a few days to one week.

The big difference between Dengue and the Zika virus is that Zika can cause significant defects in the unborn child of a pregnant woman. Zika is thought to trigger microcephaly, leading to underdeveloped heads and brains. This has only recently appeared in significant numbers, particularly in Brazil. Doctors suspect that the Zika virus has mutated to cause this new health problem during pregnancy, or it may only affect those who have had Dengue Fever and then contracted Zika during pregnancy.

Another complication associated only with the Zika virus is temporary paralysis due to Guillain-Barré Syndrome.

Anyone who is pregnant and feels unwell up to two weeks after being in an area where Zika is reported should contact a doctor immediately and report the possibility of having Zika.

Those who are pregnant should protect themselves from mosquito bites and if possible avoid visiting Zika-infected areas including the South Pacific, Hawaii, Brazil, Africa, SE Asia, South and Central America.

In healthy individuals, Zika usually causes mild illness and few people need hospital treatment or die. Unlike Dengue, Zika does not create the risk of hemorrhagic fever. Once a person has had Zika, they are protected from the disease thereafter.

Only a blood test can accurately diagnose Zika form Dengue. There is currently no vaccine or medication for either. Sufferers of Zika are advised to rest, drink plenty of fluids, use paracetamol or acetaminophen to reduce the fever and pain and avoid taking aspirin, ibuprofen or NSAIDS just in case it is Dengue Fever and may cause internal bleeding.

Symptoms of Dengue Fever

As shown earlier in the book, the symptoms and timing of Dengue Fever vary from one person to another. For most people, the first symptoms are:

- Sudden onset of a high fever
- Nausea
- Vomiting
- Severe headache

However, these common symptoms can also be the first signs of many other less serious diseases such as Zika, influenza or a viral infection. The only way to confirm whether or not you have Dengue Fever is through a blood test.

Other symptoms of Dengue Fever are:

- Diarrhea
- Bleeding gums or nose
- Fatigue

More serious symptoms include:

- Low white blood cell count
- Leakage of plasma from the blood vessels
- Depletion of fluid from the circulation

In the most severe cases Dengue Fever may cause:

- Organ dysfunction
- Internal bleeding
- Slow heart rate
- Inflammation of the brain
- Acute liver failure

The fever usually abates after a few days and is followed by a skin rash which appears 3-6 days after the first symptoms. The rash is usually bright red and the spots do not disappear when the skin is pressed. The rash is very fine and bumpy, similar to measles.

In the case of both myself and my husband, the rash slowly drained downwards as it receded from the top to the bottom of the legs. It looked like red knee-high socks, then ankle socks, then it lingered around the edges of the feet.

The hands and feet also become very tender, red and inflamed. It is difficult to walk or even be in contact with anything solid or hard such as shoes or tile flooring.

Treatment of Dengue Fever

There is no currently no vaccine, treatment or cure for Dengue Fever or Zika; doctors can only treat the symptoms.

Pain relievers are used to lower the fever and help with pain relief. Both acetaminophen and paracetamol are suitable but any painkillers containing aspirin or ibuprofen should be avoided. They thin the blood which can be very dangerous as Dengue Fever causes blood vessels and capillaries to leak fluid. The leakage can lead to a failure of the circulatory system and shock, which can be fatal. This coupled with low platelets makes internal hemorrhaging extremely serious.

Keeping the patient cool while the fever persists is very important. Sponge the body, face and neck with a cool flannel or use a shower or pool to cool off. The

Frogg Togg Chilly Pad is invaluable for applying a cool compress to the forehead, neck and chest during this stage of the fever.

Make sure the patient drinks plenty of fluids to prevent dehydration. In some cases fluid replacement may be necessary.

Doctors may prescribe anti-emetics for the nausea and vomiting.

Rest and sleep are nature's way of helping the body fight the infection.

Complications of Dengue Fever

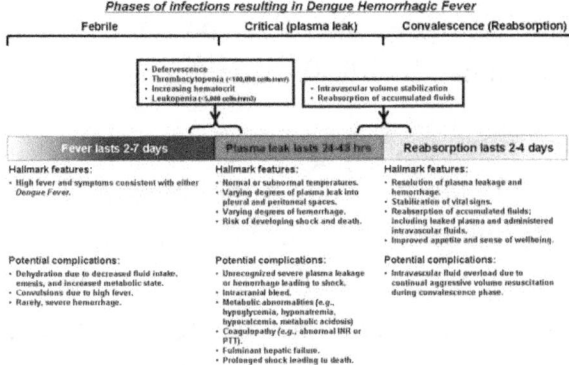

A secondary infection of Dengue Fever is likely to be far more serious and may lead to Viral Hemorrhagic Fever (VHF). This is characterized by a high fever, nausea, a rash, low white blood cell count and internal bleeding.

Once the fever declines, the infection enters the critical phase when Hemorrhagic Fever causes the blood vessels to become more permeable, leaking fluid into the peritoneum and pleural cavity between the lungs. This loss of fluid can cause a drop in blood pressure, failure of the circulatory system and Dengue Shock Syndrome (DSS), which can be life-threatening.

In more severe infections, the virus affects the liver and bone marrow. If the stromal cells in the bone marrow are affected, this lowers the platelet count in the blood which means there is greater risk of hemorrhaging coupled with poor blood clotting.

Complications of Zika Virus

For most people the Zika virus is far less serious than Dengue Fever, with few complications. The only exception to this is if the Zika sufferer is pregnant, when Zika can cause underdevelopment of the head and brain of the unborn fetus.

How to Avoid Dengue Fever

Hopefully a vaccine will shortly be available to immunize people at risk, particularly those who live in developing countries or have already had the infection once. Various companies are running clinical trials or have vaccines at the pre-clinical stage of development.

In the meantime, the best way to avoid Dengue Fever and Zika is by avoiding places where Aedes mosquitos live and breed. The mosquitos commonly inhabit tree holes, plants, flowerpots and containers where rainwater collects. They also inhabit water storage containers, rain gutters, pet water bowls, bird baths, storm drains, septic tanks, wells and even sink/shower drains and toilets.

Aedes mosquitos lay their eggs just above the waterline and once the rain floods the eggs with water the larvae hatch. It takes just seven days for the eggs to become adults and each mosquito has a lifespan of around three weeks.

Responsible householders and governments control mosquitos through insecticide spraying around the home and garden and emptying any containers that collect water.

On a personal level, using a repellant containing DEET or lemon eucalyptus can reduce the risk of being bitten by a mosquito. Covering up is helpful, especially in the first two hours of the morning and in the evening before sunset when the mosquitos are most active. Wear long sleeved shirts, long pants and socks and cover infant carriers, cribs and strollers with mosquito netting.

Homes should have screens on windows and doors to allow breezes in but keep mosquitos out.

Conclusion

I certainly did not expect the after-effects of Dengue Fever to be so long-lasting or disabling. The painful joints and inflammation lingered long after the fever had gone. At times I wondered what had happened to my health and mobility as it had deteriorated so much. I also feared that I was getting severe arthritis in my joints, but research reassured me that it was all a normal part of getting over Dengue Fever.

I hope this day-by-day account helps other sufferers to know what to expect through each phase of Dengue Fever. Hopefully my research and personal experience, along with the parallel account of my husband's symptoms, will lessen your levels of anxiety about your health if you are unfortunate enough to contract this tropical virus.

In the meantime, note the warning that getting Dengue Fever a second time can be far more serious, and even fatal. The best way to avoid such a risk is to do your research and stay away from any country in the tropics and the subtropics where Dengue Fever is prevalent until a proven vaccine is available.

Further Information Sources

World Health Organization (WHO)
http://www.who.int/mediacentre/facts
heets/fs117/en/

US Centers for Disease Control and
Prevention (CDC)
http://www.cdc.gov/dengue/
http://wwwnc.cdc.gov/travel/yellowbo
ok/2014/chapter-3-infectious-
diseases-related-to-travel/dengue

Australian Government Department
of Health
http://www.health.gov.au/internet/mai
n/publishing.nsf/Content/cda-surveil-
nndss-casedefs-cd_dengue.htm

UK National Health Service (NHS)
http://www.nhs.uk/Conditions/dengue
/Pages/Symptoms.aspx

UK Know Before You Go NHS
https://www.gov.uk/knowbeforeyougo

UK Hospital for Tropical Diseases
http://www.thehtd.org/

UK Gov. Foreign travel Advice
http://www.fitfortravel.nhs.uk/home.aspx

UK Health Advice for World Cup
Brazil 2014
https://www.gov.uk/government/news/health-advice-for-fans-heading-to-brazil-for-the-world-cup

Public Health Agency of Canada
(PHAC)
http://www.phac-aspc.gc.ca/tmp-pmv/notices-avis/index-eng.php